Christ Defeats Cancer 2
The Battle Continues

Christ Defeats Cancer 2:
The Battle Continues

by

Scotty McCoy

with editing by

Sarah Snyder

and a foreword written by

Dr. Na Tosha Gatson

Published by Gravestone Publishing

ISBN-13: 978-1720858201
ISBN-10: 1720858209

THIS BOOK CONTINUES TO TELL THE STORY AND JOURNEY OF MY DAD, SCOTT G. MCCOY, AS HE CONTINUES HIS BATTLE WITH GLIOBLASTOMA. SINCE *CHRIST DEFEATS CANCER*, HE HAS HAD SIDE EFFECTS, MINOR COMPLICATIONS, AND ULTIMATE TRIUMPHS THAT, THROUGH FAITH AND PRAYER, ULTIMATELY ALLOWED SCOTT G. MCCOY TO BE VICTORIOUS, YET MORE IMPORTANTLY, ALLOWED JESUS CHRIST TO TRIUMPH IN VICTORY. MY DAD IS STILL CANCER FREE THANKS TO OUR LORD AND SAVIOR. I LOVE YOU DAD! KEEP WINNING THE BATTLE AND FIGHTING THE FIGHT!

ACKNOWLEDGEMENTS

The Family: Thanks to both the McCoy and Seitzinger families for going through this long, exhausting, and emotional journey with us. We got through this together as a family and I know it wasn't easy, but by God's grace and strength we did it!

Our Friends: I want to thank our family friends for being there for us throughout our time of need. Even though things are looking up and everyt hing is going the way God has planned, our friends continue to be a great source of support. They helped us tremendously when we needed them the most. We thank you from the bottom of our hearts.

My Publisher: I want to thank my publisher, Tanya Ballinger, who has helped me in more ways than I could ever repay her. She has gone above and beyond her duties of senior publisher for KDP.

Jesus Christ: And I saved the best for last. Thanks to our Lord and Savior, Jesus Christ. Because of Him, my dad survived the toughest fight of his life. Jesus provided the miracle for my dad to beat cancer. As the Bible states: "Through Jesus stripes, my dad is healed."

ABOUT THE AUTHOR

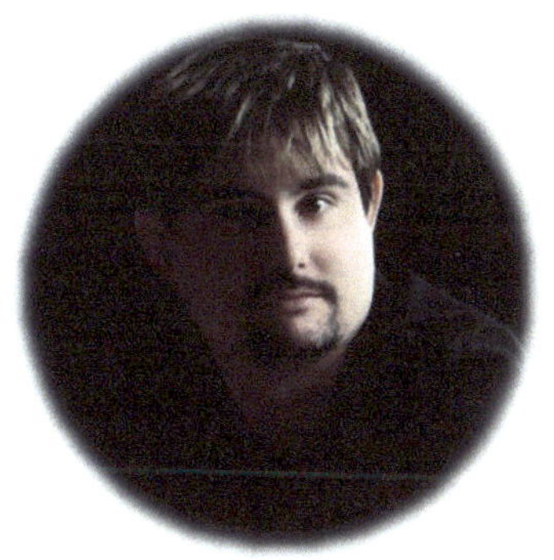

I, Scotty McCoy, was born on December 6, 1989. I am a published author, who has accomplished a lot in my young adult life.

I obtained an Associate's of Applied Science Degree from *Luzerne County Community College* in Web/Software Development and a Bachelor of Science Degree from *Champlain College* in Web/Software Development, as well as a specialized certification in Computer Science from the South Campus of *Schuylkill Technology Centers*. Despite my educational accomplishments, I am not shy in learning, educating, and challenging myself in new subjects, ventures, and endeavors.

I graduated in 2008 from *North Schuylkill Jr./Sr. High School*. I had a teacher named Mrs. Joann Hoppel for English class in 9th and 12th grades. I stated in various interviews, that because of the knowledge obtained in her classes; I retrieved the skills and confidence needed to become a successful author.

I have published four books: *The Ultimate Friday the 13th Trivia Book*, *The Ultimate Halloween Trivia Book*, *Christ Defeats Cancer*, which has officially made the New York Times Bestsellers List, and *The Ultimate Halloween Trivia Book, 2nd Edition*. This is my fifth book; a sequel to *Christ Defeats Cancer*, which continues my dad's journey with fighting the wretched disease of brain cancer, as well as diving more into scripture and what this cancer is and how truly horrid of a disease it is: *Christ Defeats Cancer 2: The Battle Continues.*

I appeared on various radio shows, podcasts, television and web series, and in magazines and on Websites as a celebrity guest to promote my career in writing, such as on the *Return to Camp Blood Radio Show*, two interviews on *Python's Paradise*, *Interviews with Everyday People*, *Klimczak's Killer Collection*, *Resurrection of Zombie Radio Show*, *Skook News*, two Christian radio stations: *WGRC* and *WPGM*, the *Horror Fuel* Website, and in the December 2016 edition of *Popcorn Horror* magazine.

My writing is mostly about the horror genre, where I write about various horror-related topics and subjects. I also had various book signings, including in Frackville, Pennsylvania at the *Whippoorwill Dam*, *Barnes and Noble* at the *King of Prussia Mall*, *Bible Depot* in Sunbury, Pennsylvania, the *AppleFest* in Ashland, Pennsylvania, the *Pioneer Tunnel* in Ashland, Pennsylvania, and the *Walk-In Art Center* in Schuylkill Haven, Pennsylvania. I also had a double event: concert/book signing, at the *New Hope Wesleyan Church* in Frackville, Pennsylvania, where I hosted the book signing and Tiffany Maley did a two-part concert.

I had various jobs, including a Software Database Engineer position at *Computer Software Incorporated*, a Senior PHP Web and Mobile Application Developer position at *GINtech Systems*, a supervisory role at *Kmart*, a cashier position at *McDonald's*, and a Web Development and Computer Information Systems Tutor, as well as a Peer Mentoring position at *Luzerne County Community College.*

I also am an online college professor at *Champlain College* where I teach both programming and theory-related courses in the Web/Software Development curriculum for the Continuing Professional Studies (CPS) department. Two courses I teach include WEBD-310 (Server-Side Scripting with PHP) and WEBD-325 (Advanced PHP Programming). I currently work for the *United States Coast Guard* as their Website Developer in the Technical Information Management Branch.

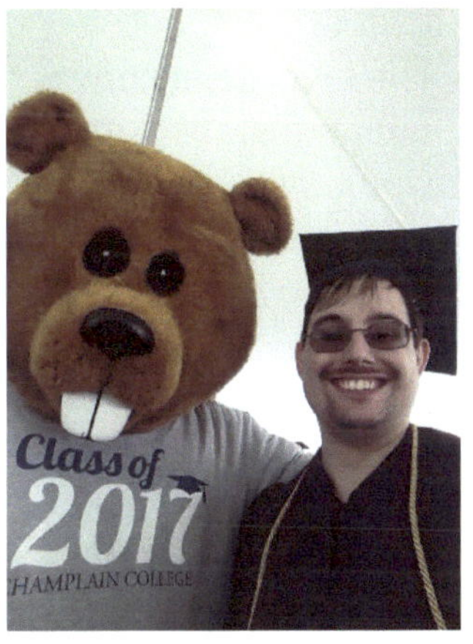

I graduated from *Champlain College* with a 3.88 GPA as a Summa Cum Laude (Latin Honors) graduate. I had the honor of being inducted into the Alpha Sigma Lambda National Honor Society; the most prestigious honor society for adult students.

I've endured a difficult childhood because of bullying, due to a diagnosis of Tourette's Syndrome. I've demonstrated to people faced with adversity that all things are possible through Christ. So, if you want to do something, just work hard, focus, and put your mind to it and your dreams can come true.

Sincerely,

Scotty McCoy

Scotty McCoy
Author and Philanthropist

ABOUT SCOTT G. MCCOY

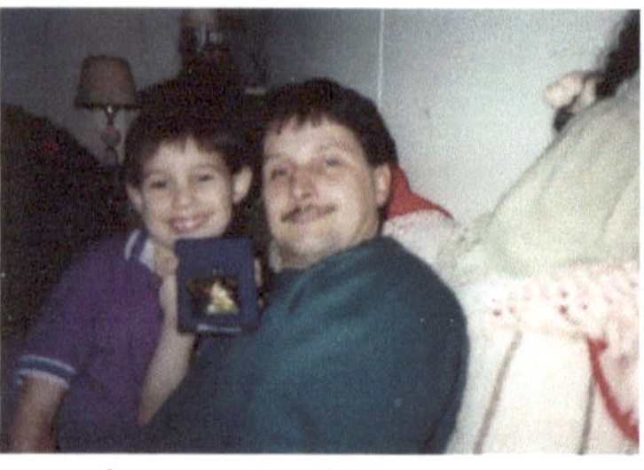 Scott McCoy was always quiet when growing up, but he was caring and would do anything for anybody. Scott enjoyed playing sports, especially baseball, and was an amazing pitcher. He always ate healthily and made a habit of using his brother, Ken's weights to work out. His favorite meal was spaghetti as a kid and it still is. My mom remembers my grandmother telling her that my dad would grow up to be a minister, as he loved going to Sunday School and church.

My dad was always a hardworking man who would do the simplest of things for anybody in need, such as unfreezing his mom's pipes during the winter months. He was the type of worker that didn't mind "getting his hands dirty" by doing manual labor work. He worked for 28 years at the Frackville, Pennsylvania state prison. He also catered on the side and has catered countless spaghetti and meatloaf dinners for Zion's Reformed United Church of Christ.

After speaking with my dad's sister, Marci; she told me a story that describes my dad's growing up years. My aunt Marci is his older sister, and she reports always tormenting and picking on him. At one point, their mom, my grandmother, told my dad, "don't ever hit girls." Marci used this to her advantage, until one day my dad said, enough was enough and he hit her back in self-defense. Marci, shocked, ran to her parents (my grandparents), and told them my dad hit her back. As Marci told me this story, I could hear my grandmother's voice as she laughed "Ah ha, ah ha, now you did it! I told you to stop picking on him, so you had it coming for not listening!" As Marci concluded the story, she told me her parents were right. She had it coming!

My dad was always concerned about other people. It was easier for him to put others before himself. He did this ever since he was a kid. His dad always told him that big boys should not cry. So, he would hold back his tears during sad moments that would happen in his life. After speaking about this topic with my aunt Marci, she encouraged him that it was okay to cry, because "real men cry." I remember when my grandfather passed away, my dad wouldn't cry, but you can tell he wanted too. The same response came when his mother and brothers, Ken and Joe, passed away.

My dad went through a lot of heartache later in his life, such as losing both of his parents and two brothers. He walks in peace; knowing they all are in Heaven with our Lord and Savior, Jesus Christ. When they all passed away, he never once cried in front of people. But, I believe he fought back tears, because it was his way of trying to show everybody he was strong.

I remember when my grandfather, who was in the hospital, passed away. While in the hospital he made me promise that when he died, I wouldn't cry. Well, he passed away and at his funeral, I bawled my eyes out. My dad saw how upset I was, so he tried to make me smile by telling a joke. My dad stated, "Didn't you promise pap you wouldn't cry when he passed away?" I responded with a whimper in my voice, "Yeah!" My dad followed up by saying "Well, you just broke that promise!" The funny thing is that his reminder put a smirk on my face and I didn't cry for the remainder of the funeral. I knew my pap wanted me to be happy and to be comforted by the fact that he was at peace and no longer suffering.

Marci told me another story about my dad, pertaining me. This shows how my dad's desire and humility in wanting me to become a man. In 1991, I was two years old. During that time, the laws weren't as strict as they are today. My dad brought me to my grandmother's house. My grandmother said to Marci, when telling the story, that my dad brought me to her house on a cool day without wearing a coat. She asked my dad, "Where is his coat?" He replied, "My son is not going to grow up to become a wimp!"

He always showed determination and we knew this was God's strength, allowing my dad to survive emergency brain surgery and a major stroke, complete radiation therapy and rehabilitation, and defeat brain cancer. The persevering mindset my dad grew up with and developed was helpful in his battle.

I had an amazing childhood and father. My father amazes me to this day. He is so strong and brave, which I believe were essential in helping him to survive brain cancer. Our Christian beliefs were instrumental in his victory and recovery as well. My dad is such an inspiration to me and my family, and hopefully to everyone who reads his success story.

His battle with cancer, which I posted on Facebook, went viral; and I hope this inspired people to believe, have faith, and stay positive. With this type of inspiration, my dad believes that other people battling cancer will discover hope and the will to fight until they achieve victory.

I don't think I could go through everything he did and survive. It has been a long two and a half years. I would be too scared to face the battle that he did, yet I sometimes wish it was me instead of him because he is an amazing gracious man. I know if it weren't for God; even watching my dad would have been impossible. But thanks to God, I could watch my dad not just fight for his life, but also survive and eventually thrive in the battle, and thus coming out on top years later.

My dad is not any ordinary person. He is a strong Christian, who permitted Jesus to overcome Satan's curse that was placed upon him and our family. Dad told my aunt Marci "I will survive this fight. I am not ready to leave my wife and son." Once again, he was thinking of others and not of himself. My dad continued, "I'm not afraid to die, I just don't want to leave my family." Family is important to my dad. He would do everything possible to maintain it.

All my dad wanted was for his friends and family to be by his side, and boy he had that. The medical staff joked about having a celebrity in the hospital, because of the huge support system he had. I jokingly said to the staff, "You do have a celebrity here! I'm a famous published author!" My dad then laughed and jokingly said "This is The Scotty McCoy Hour" which he often said, when I talked about myself because of my ego. HA!

Two days after the surgery, my dad had the stroke. He was in the Intensive Care Unit (ICU). Even though his life was hanging by a thread, he was still thinking of others before himself. He asked Marci if she could order Centiole's, a famous local pizza place known for their homemade pizza pies, to serve the nurses. He also asked Marci to order my mom flowers.

During his recovery, his determination was to get well. He had amazing nurses, including Julie and Heather, both of whom he talks about to this day. He cannot thank them enough for how well they did their job nursing him back to health. He surprised and amazed the entire medical team at Geisinger Medical Center in Danville, Pennsylvania about how fast he was recovering and getting back on his feet.

Various family members and even friends told him, "Scott, you have helped so many people in your life. It is now time for us to be able to give back to you." Even though my dad didn't like hearing those words, and often resisted us when we would do something for him that he wanted to do, he appreciated the love and support from his family and friends. He eventually got used to it. Although he had no choice in the matter. HA!

Since *Christ Defeats Cancer* was published and this sequel has been written and published, two and a half years has officially gone by, and I, as his son, still cry myself to sleep some nights after thinking of the suffering that my dad went through and how his life has changed. I still have nightmares on a nightly basis. This made me realize that life is too short and never to take it for granted. Don't just tell your loved ones that you love them but show them because you never know when they'll take their last breath or something tragic, sudden, and unexpected can happen and change your life.

At the time of diagnosis, my dad was only 54 years old. Too young to have something like this happen to him, so you never know when something can happen. Just realize that in a blink of an eye, your life can change forever. You are never too young to die or to get a life-threatening condition. Thankfully, my dad is still alive, and I will never take him for granted like I used to.

To this day, I look at my dad and want to cry, even as I am writing this. I realize in the moment, I almost lost my father. But as the fighter that he is, and through the perseverance and power given to him by our Lord Jesus Christ, Glioblastoma has been defeated.

One thing cancer has learned through this entire battle was that when you come face to face with Christ, you stand no chance of winning. As Scott McCoy's spirit has been filled with the undying love and purity of our Lord Jesus and His divine healing; Satan has been defeated once again. Amen!

THE PREDECESSOR

Christ Defeats Cancer did amazing in the selling department and has reached worldwide fame and acknowledgement. It has captured the eyes of celebrities, such as Robin Roberts from Good Morning America, Adam Marcus, who directed *Jason Goes to Hell: The Final Friday*, and even Lana Parrilla, whom I mentioned it to at the *Once Upon a Time* convention and she has posted about it on Twitter and Instagram. I think out of them all, Lana Parrilla is my all-time favorite to acknowledge it because, no offense to the others and everyone else, but she is my favorite actress on my favorite show.

Within 35-minutes of its initial release, *Christ Defeats Cancer* grossed over $2000 in sales and sold well over 100 copies alone from people worldwide, including all over the United States of America, Canada, the United Kingdom, Australia, and Germany. My publisher, Tanya Ballinger, was thrilled with its sales in just 35-minutes of publication that a sequel was immediately approved and here comes *Christ Defeats Cancer 2: The Battle Continues.*

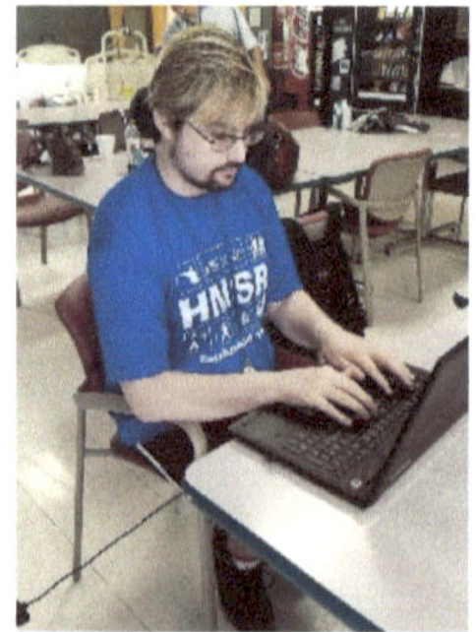

Not to get into the major plot points of the interior from this novel, but this book was primarily written on visits I made with my dad at the HealthSouth rehabilitation facility located outside of Geisinger Medical Center in Danville, Pennsylvania. And boy it was fun, tiring, depressing, and interesting to say the least to write a sequel to a book that brought back so many horrible, yet some amazing memories that we had to suffer and sustain from as a family the past two plus years.

Christ Defeats Cancer, the predecessor of *Christ Defeats Cancer 2: The Battle Continues*, had numerous book signings, autograph sessions, meet and greets, testimonies, support group discussions, photo ops, and tons of publicity. *Christ Defeats Cancer* was even added to the *New York Times Best Seller's List*, which is a rarity for independently published novels. I will mention, if you hadn't purchased or read *Christ Defeats Cancer*, then you must do that before you can even begin to read this one, so you can be caught up on the events that had transpired to get to where we are as a family today. Upon reading *Christ Defeats Cancer*, you'll know the trials and tribulations that occurred from day one of diagnosis and conclude with the present day in this sequel.

For *Christ Defeats Cancer*, I have had book signings at *Bible Depot*, a bookstore located in Sunbury, Pennsylvania, *New Hope Wesleyan Church* in Frackville, Pennsylvania, Pioneer Tunnel in Ashland, Pennsylvania, Christmas Pines Campground in Auburn, Pennsylvania, Eureka Park in Ashland, Pennsylvania, Renninger's Farmer's Market in Orwigsburg, Pennsylvania, and the Walk In Art Center in Schuylkill Haven, Pennsylvania. I even did a meet and greet at the Rolling Meadows Clubhouse in Lavelle, Pennsylvania for *Christ Defeats Cancer*. To date, I sold a rough estimate of over $5000 in royalties, maybe even more than that, and counting. There are also future book signings in the works, and there will be tons of events I'll be conducting for the foreseeable future regarding *Christ Defeats Cancer*.

If you need hope, inspiration, encouragement, belief, faith, love, restoration, or anything at all in your battle or a loved one's battle with cancer, *Christ Defeats*

Cancer is a must read for you. In doing so, you'll bear witness to a true, real life miracle that I, along with my mom, dad, and entire family and even family friends have witnessed. Dr. Toms, who wrote the foreword to *Christ Defeats Cancer* even stated from his own mouth that it was a true miracle that science cannot explain.

So, get *Christ Defeats Cancer*, if you already haven't done so, and then read this and bear witness to a true miracle performed from the Almighty Lord and Savior, Jesus Christ, with both books being told about the living miracle, Scott George McCoy, told from the point of view of his son, the author, Scotty McCoy, with bits and pieces inserted from the McCoy and Seitzinger families. Come join us on the journey and praise the Lord for his miraculous and supernatural work he has done for my dad. Let us rejoice, celebrate, and revel in the glory of God. Amen!

FOREWORD

Many Directions of GBM Treatment:
Arms **outstretched**, to reach out and grab hold of loved ones near and afar and for the treatments we know to exist. With a grateful spirit, we look **back** to appreciate the distance we have travelled and the knowledge of our own mistakes and miracles. We lean **in** to pull on the strengths that we are made of in order to move **onward** with the fight for quality. We go **down** to our knees and send prayers **up** for the spiritual strength that sustains us each day. I have learned that there are so many places we need to look for treatment, and most of those cannot be prescribed.

As a Neuro-Oncologist – I am not just limited to use of the medical therapies available in a neurosurgical suite, a radiation center, and a pharmacy to treat glioblastoma (GBM). I have learned that I must also rely on the patient, the family, and the entire spiritual support system that uplifts my patient. This book offers information that demonstrates the many directions our patients and their families must go in order to find

The Physician
I am a Physician-Scientist of trained in neuro-oncology and neuroimmunology, and I currently serve as the Director of Neuro-Oncology at Geisinger Health in Pennsylvania. I completed my undergraduate training at Indiana University, then attended The Ohio State University to complete a MD and PhD, as well as a neurology residency and a post-doctoral research year within the Department of Neurosurgery. I then spent two-years as part of a neuro-oncology fellowship with the University of Texas MD Anderson Cancer Center.

I am a mother of three and friends describe me as a compassionate motivator. I am often asked, "How do you work in such an emotionally draining career such as brain cancer?" My reply… I am often inspired by the victorious spirit of my patient population who focuses on taking from each day the maximum amount of GOOD.

My patients seem to recognize that long life is less important than quality life – and that quality is determined differently by different patients and patient families. I learn from my patients that life is actually long (as it is the longest thing that we as humans will ever do), and that the parts of life that are truly short are the times we have with our loved ones, enjoying good health, and the time we spend in our careers.

My patients have taught me to help focus on improving these parts of their lives – and in-turn, I focus on improving those parts in my own life. I gain wisdom, peace, comfort, and a spirit of gratitude from each patient encounter. Getting to know and work with patients like Mr. McCoy and his family are valued pieces of my life and my career that keep me encouraged.

I am honored to write this foreword and share in telling the story of a victorious spirit who has leaned on his providers, himself, his family, and his God to bring about a treatment plan of care and outcome that serves as his personal testimony for the human condition.

What is GBM?
Last year, nearly 79,000 people were diagnosed with primary brain tumors in the US. Glioblastoma (GBM) has an incidence of about 3.5 cases per 100,000 people in the U.S. and more common in Caucasian males over age 60.

GBM is the deadliest and most common of primary brain tumor in adults with the median overall survival of less than 16 months even with standard of care surgery, radiation, and chemotherapy.

Despite many years of research, only two treatments have been approved by the FDA for newly diagnosed GBM to improve survival in the past nearly 15 years. An estimated 5% of patients with the diagnosis survive at 5-years and use of tumor treating fields medical device improves the patient survival to only 13% at 5 years when used in combination with the standard of care therapy.

Disease progression is virtually inevitable, and effective second-line therapies are limited, thus, early detection and rapid clinical judgement are needed to determine next treatment steps. There are a limited number of safe neurosurgical and radiation interventions available at the time of GBM progression, and the natural history of GBM is to develop resistance to medical therapies. Clinical decline impacts quality of life and limits the clinician's choice for new and potentially poorly tolerated anti-tumor therapies.

Goals are to control tumor progression, identify and treat progression early, and work to maintain patient dignity and quality of live while extending overall survival. This is a high-grade primary brain tumor that is difficult to treat at onset.

The Clinical Story of Mr. Scott McCoy:
On December 14, 2018, Scotty contacted me to write the foreword to his book and give a little insight on Glioblastoma and the entire backstory, in a nutshell, of his father's condition and progress as he battled Glioblastoma.

With permission from Scotty, his mother, his father, and the rest of the family, I have been honored to accept writing this entire foreword and will conclude it by giving a brief history regarding Mr. Scott McCoy's journey these past few years.

At age 54, (Sept. 2016), Mr. McCoy presented to the emergency room with worsening fatigue, balance, confusion, leg weakness, and headaches. Imaging of his brain revealed an aggressive appearing right-sided brain tumor. The decision to go forward with brain surgery, with a highly talented and well-respected neurosurgeon, was made and everyone awaited the outcome. The pathology was returned as GBM and his journey began. Mr. McCoy a underwent brain irradiation given with chemotherapy, then followed with 12 additional cycles of adjuvant chemotherapy and use of the TTF device through most of 2017.

Just before Christmas 2017, I inherited the care of Mr. McCoy and continue close surveillance and monitoring until progression in March of 2018. We opted for additional oral chemotherapy with additional focused brain radiation therapy at that time. Mr. McCoy uses the Optune TTF device greater than average 70% of the time throughout the ups and downs of his treatment.

By August 2018, he suffered some motor decline suspected due to brain swelling. We added a biologic agent useful to help with reducing inflammation as well as limiting the development of new blood vessels that might be supplying the brain tumor. Noting persistently low platelets on oral chemotherapy, our team decided to discontinue these agents and switch to immunotherapies, which are currently at the center of multiple clinical trials ongoing in the field. Without too much of an insurance battle, the patient was approved to start immunotherapy in combination with the biologic agent, both tolerated well.

Our most recent visit with Mr. McCoy, peaceful, grateful and surrounded by enthusiastic family – presented with left arm and leg weakness and slightly elevated blood pressure. MRI brain with perfusion remains stable without evidence of progression in March of 2019… Two years and six months after diagnosis of GBM.

I gain wisdom, peace, comfort, and a spirit of gratitude from each patient encounter. Getting to know and work with patients like Mr. McCoy and his family are valued pieces of my life and my career that shield me from *burn-out*. I am honored to write this foreword and share in telling the story of the victorious Mr. Scott McCoy who has leaned on his providers, himself, his family, and his God to bring about a comprehensive treatment plan and an uncommon outcome that serves as his personal testimony for the human condition.

Sincerely,

Na Tosha N. Gatson

Na Tosha N. Gatson, MD, PhD
Physician-Scientist
Neuro-Oncology and Neuroimmunology
Assistant Professor of Research & Clinical Medicine

INTRODUCTION

In *Christ Defeats Cancer*, we used the following six words to describe what life is and which proper characteristics are a true sentiment on what describes my father, Scott George McCoy: faith, strength, perseverance, determination, love, and survivor. Moving on a few years later after the initial diagnosis and battle with Glioblastoma, these words still ring true. However, here is a new puzzle to solve: what do the following six words represent:

Miracle	Courageous
Fighter	Brave
Stubborn	Godly

The words above can all be summed up with one simple sentence: *A fighter of cancer, but a survivor of cancer*. Yes, stubborn is included in that last! You must be stubborn to keep fighting and battling cancer, so you don't let cancer win, and one thing we all know about my dad is that he is the most stubborn man I know, which isn't a bad thing.

So, Scott George McCoy is a survivor of cancer due to his possession of the following character traits: faith, strength, perseverance, determination, love, survivor, miracle, fighter, stubborn, courageous, brave, and Godly. Those twelve words are what describe a true hero, inspiration, and cancer survivor. And as his son, my dad is my hero. He is my inspiration. He is my life. He made me want to become a philanthropist and brain cancer awareness activist. I never knew how bad this disease was, until I personally seen my dad struggle.

In *Christ Defeats Cancer*, my dad's story was told. In *Christ Defeats Cancer 2: The Battle Continues*, my dad's story is continued. This continuing battle doesn't necessarily mean a loss of the battle or major complications. It simply means the continuing battle with Glioblastoma is foretold in a way that no one has heard.

It'll give updates on my dad's progress from where the original story left off. It'll give updates on any minor complications, all doctor appointments, any struggles and challenges, various side effects, the ultimate triumphs my dad has had since the telling of his original battle, and the expansion on what Glioblastoma is with an in-depth, full on chapter of this horrid disease to make those unaware of this awful form of brain cancer aware of how bad it is and what my dad must deal with on a daily and hourly basis. Plus, the inclusion of various scriptures told by the Lord and to encourage, give even more hope, love, and faith to those in need, and to even show everyone that a one to two-year survival rate given to my dad is not a death sentence because my dad's over two years and still hasn't seen a reformation of the tumor.

Get ready for this tale because the bumpy ride told in *Christ Defeats Cancer* gets an upgrade. The bumpy ride will continue in *Christ Defeats Cancer 2: The Battle Continues* with a more spiritual, Christian view of Jesus' love. It'll give those who have lost faith in the Lord a restoration in his miraculous and supernatural power. It'll give those who have lost hope in defeating cancer the hope to survive cancer. It'll give those who don't believe in miracles the foretold proof of our Lord and Savior, Jesus Christ, being a true miracle worker.

As previously stated, *Christ Defeats Cancer* is getting an upgrade. Most sequels don't follow up to the hype of the original, however, *Christ Defeats Cancer 2: The Battle Continues* goes above and beyond and you are about to see the true power of the Lord and how he continues to help my dad cope, fight, and defeat cancer.

TABLE OF CONTENTS

PREVIOUSLY IN *CHRIST DEFEATS CANCER*

My dad and I had a huge fight on September 6, 2016 at a Seitzinger family reunion. I never apologized to him regarding the fight, but figured it was no big deal and nothing would come of it. I mean, it was just a little father-son tiff, we'd have plenty more to come and plenty of time to make up after the tension blows over. But I didn't realize what was going to happen in the forthcoming month.

It was around the time my dad and I went on a bus trip with the Gordon, Pennsylvania Boy Scouts Troop to Washington DC that he began showing signs and symptoms of something unidentified and unknown to anyone. As previously spoken about in *Christ Defeats Cancer*, we thought my dad was just being his goofy self at first, or just wasn't really paying attention to his every move. Dropping pickle jars in Wal Mart to forgetting to put on his pants when going to go to the store to driving incoherently to and from various locations by going through stop signs and red lights, going over to the other side of the road, and just not paying attention to his surroundings while driving. The latter, scaring both myself and my mom, because we were both unaware of what could have happened to not just us, but to other drivers on the road due to my dad's reckless driving.

It came down to taking my dad to the Shamokin Hospital after his good friend, John, called my mom and telling her that we need to rush my dad to the hospital as he isn't acting like his true self. My dad worked with John as a landscaper for the state of Pennsylvania (PennDOT) after retirement from the Frackville State Prison.

As my mom rushed up from my aunt Lou Ann's house, with whom she was visiting when receiving the phone call from John, my dad wasn't home. She is asking me in a stern, concerned tone of voice where my dad's at. I'm sitting on the couch surfing Facebook, as I always do from my laptop, yelling at her to tell me what's the matter. I know my dad drove down to the church where he has his Boy Scout meetings, but I was unsure if he was in a car accident. She then told me what John said via the aforementioned phone call.

My dad came home, as my aunt Lou Ann, uncle Steve, my mom, and I waited for him to come into the living room. We sat him on the couch and my uncle did a simple examination on him. Upon examining him, he agreed something didn't look right so we rushed him to the hospital. Steve thought it was nothing less than a tick bite affecting him and nothing more than a possible mini stroke. But we never expected the diagnosis we first received.

Not doing proper testing, they released my dad with a simple diagnosis of dehydration. They filled him up with fluids and let him go home. Steve wasn't satisfied with such a diagnosis, and in return, did some online research, using his medical experience he has as a physician assistant, to determine that it was something more neurological. Steve did some neurological testing on my dad, as well as myself and my mom.

He showed us that my mom and I have a properly function brain, so to speak. However, my dad failed the test which means something in his brain isn't working properly, which still leads us to think it was a tick bite (causing symptoms of Lyme Disease) or even a mini stroke. We knew it wasn't a major stroke or my dad wouldn't be able to move or even speak. But whatever it was needed to be addressed and we rushed my dad back to the Shamokin Hospital for retesting, and this time, Steve and myself made sure the hospital staff did their job properly by doing a CT Scan. I even told them, "You are lucky we aren't pressing charges for an improper diagnosis and lack of patient care due to us knowing that something is happening inside my dad's brain due to neurological tests we provided ourselves." The nurses looked at me, dumbfounded with a concerned look, knowing what they have done could've been a result of life or death.

They did the proper testing this time and the CT Scan showed that my dad had a large mass (otherwise known as a tumor) on the brain. It was uncertain what kind of tumor it was. It was unsure if it was cancerous or not. However, they were going to rush my dad via an ambulance to the main unit of Geisinger Medical Center in Danville, Pennsylvania.

Upon hearing the diagnosis of my dad's brain tumor, my mom was completely silenced. Not a tear shed as she was in complete and utter shock. She couldn't believe what she heard. I, on the other hand, screamed. I started crying and shouting aloud in a hysterical tone of voice. My body buckled. My legs became shaky and wobbly. I felt as if I was floating on thin air. It all felt like a bad dream that I wouldn't wake up from. As I screamed, my body buckling, and my legs almost giving out, my uncle held me in his arms and told me that the tumor was operable not inoperable, so he can still beat this. All I could think of was how I have been horribly treating my dad lately, and I'd do anything to take this pain away from him.

Even when my dad was in the hospital, the night before surgery, I was talking to him as he slept, and mom was in the waiting room, telling him that I'd take this tumor from him in a heartbeat. I even prayed to God, and still do to this day every night before I sleep, for God to cure my dad and if someone must have what he does, let it be me. I'd rather suffer with what my dad does than have a good, decent human being like him deal with such a horrific disease.

God has a plan for giving it to my dad, but I pray that he'd use said plan to heal my dad and make my body the vessel. I still, to this day, argue with my dad and yell at him. I guess that's how I tolerate the pain I feel with what my dad is going through. I can't take seeing him suffering like he does, even though he does good nowadays, but I just cannot help but yell at him, my mom, or anyone else. It's two years of pain and frustration being unleashed and a daily basis of seeing my dad and being constantly reminded with how he has this dreaded, horrible disease.

My mom would come into the room with me and we'd sit next to my dad's bedside. We pulled an all-nighter. I mean who can sleep when they are awaiting the MRI results of the person you love and are unsure if the tumor is benign or cancerous. So much anxiousness and so much worry going through your mind and body. Your soul can only be soothed by praying to the Lord. My faith at the time wasn't as strong as it is now so even when I prayed, I had doubts I'd live to my 30th birthday with my dad in my life. It was a horrible feeling thinking that your own father would die at such a young age due to the enemy (otherwise known as Satan) attacking your thoughts.

I remember vividly to this day, my uncle Steve drove me to Geisinger when dad was being transported and I am praying in such an inaudible tone that only the Lord can hear as my lips quivered while I cried, and the tears trickled down my cheeks. I felt the fear coming from Satan. I felt the fear trembling throughout my body, as it made me close to the stages of hyperventilation. But this was the moment in time that I had no choice but to put my trust and faith in the Lord. I used this moment to change my life, put all of my faith in the Lord, and let it be in His hands. I had to let him be the one to show us the way and defeat Satan and the horrible curse he put upon my dad. I knew the Lord would overrule the evil Satan unleashed, and in doing so, my first of many prayers in the forthcoming months were answered: conquering fear.

Morning came around and it was 6:00 AM. Dr. Steven Toms, the neurosurgeon who was going to perform the operation on my dad, had the MRI results and it was time for the moment of truth. We found out my dad has a rare, aggressive form of brain cancer known as Glioblastoma. Not to go into much detail on the horridly horrific disease, as that is described in detail in chapter one, but this type of cancer is classified as incurable and is the deadliest form of cancer known to man. This type of cancer will keep growing back. However, by Jesus' stripes, my dad is healed. Yes, we know Jesus will do everything to heal my dad, and whatever is in His will, shall be done.

My dad was being prepped for surgery, and I called the entire family as they all slowly, but surely came into the waiting room of the main lobby. Among those in attendance was, of course, my mom and me. Then there was my aunts Lou Ann, Lesley, Marci, Candi, and Jeannette. My uncles Kirk, Ron, Joey, Dave, and Steve were also present. My cousins, Jennifer, David and his wife, Amanda, and Matthew were there for moral support as well. On top of that, we had family friends, Chrissy Korn and her mom, Darlene, Lisa Sharp and Kenny

Tregembo, my dad's good friends, John and Dan, as well as
Pastors Mark.

       We led in a prayer circle while the surgery was
taking place, led by Pastor Mark, my uncle Steve, and my
aunt Jeannette. As they were praying, everyone in the
hospital lobby agreed. We showed our agreement with the
prayer by saying "Amen." Throughout the prayer, I was
screaming. I was vocally and audibly speaking in tongues
that only the Lord, Jesus Christ, could understand what I
was saying. Praying, pleading to the Lord to let my dad
survive such a major type of surgery on an important part
of the body. My aunt Marci put her arms around the back
of my neck, as I am screaming out to the Lord, and she
whispered in my ear "Your dad is a fighter. He'll be fine. I
promise you this, buddy." Words I still hear to this day, as
clear as anything. Words that weren't just meaningful to
me but were completely true with the end results.

       After about seven or eight hours of surgery on a
cancerous tumor that was the size of a man's fist, Dr. Toms
came out to the lobby and asked if everyone is present. I,
shaking in anxiousness and wondering what exactly was
happening and if my dad is even alive, realized my aunts
Lou Ann and Lesley were missing. Leave it to those two to
be shopping in a hospital gift shop. LOL. In the end, I got
them, and they ran to the lobby. I never saw my aunt Lou
Ann run so fast before. LOL. However, after they got
back to the lobby, Dr. Toms gave us the fortunate news.
He and his team of surgeons removed 95 to 99 percent of
the tumor and the surgery was a success. I breathed a sigh
of relief and realized we're in the clear now. But boy was I
wrong.

       Two days after surgery, my dad suffered a major
stroke. I knew that he wasn't acting as himself, and the day

prior he was his goofy self and telling corny jokes. But a day after, he couldn't talk, his arm kept twitching, he couldn't keep awake. Yes, the doctors told us he'd have good and bad days, but this wasn't just a "bad day." I ordered the nurses to give my dad an emergency MRI, to which they at first declined until I put my cocky, arrogant attitude I tend to possess when I don't get my way to good use and in the end, he had the MRI done.

A good family friend, Lynn Wetzel, was sitting with my mom and I in the cafeteria eating. Granted, I barely ate a thing for roughly three days at this point and slept maybe thirty minutes the past three days, got a phone call from one of the nurses. We rushed up and they told us that they'll be taking my dad to the Intensive Care Unit as he has suffered a stroke. They couldn't tell us much more, but we'd know more information in the forthcoming days.

That Sunday, the entire family slept overnight in the waiting room as we were told my dad most likely wasn't going to survive the stroke. He was in a medically-induced coma to let his brain rest up. My uncle Steve had a vision that the Jesus put his hand inside my dad's brain and pinched the bleed to stop it. The bleeding within the brain stopped and voila, the miracle has happened. Something we never thought would come true. Something my uncle Steve told my mom and I, yet we never expected it to actually come true. Hard times, especially in life and death situations, allows easy access for Satan to have his "fun" and play torturous games on our minds and emotions.

Come Monday, they did another MRI because they needed to see if the brain bleed got worse or better. In doing so, they would need to do another brain surgery to alleviate the swelling. In short, it would prevent his brains from hitting his skull and basically exploding, so to speak, and thus killing him in the process.

The results of that MRI came back, and Dr. Toms came in with the entire family and told us that it is the strangest thing. The first MRI showed a clear sign of a stroke occurring. The second MRI showed no signs of any stroke within the brain, however, he did have the physical ailments of a stroke, as well as the surrounding cancer cells that were lit up on the first MRI being completely obliterated from the second MRI. Dr. Toms said to my mom "Your husband…" and then looks at me and says, "Your father..." and then he continues saying "Is nothing less than a miracle and nothing more than a survivor. Science cannot explain what we just witnessed." He then told us that my dad was awaking from his medically-induced coma on his own, to which I went in, gave him a hug, and now it was time to let the road to recovery process begin, but we had some snags here and there.

My dad ended up having a UTI, which he had gotten from the catheter they had to use on him. That was a frightening experience for sure because I walked in on my every five-minute visit with him and just see him convulsing, but it was due to being cold (thanks to the UTI) and not a seizure, as they initially thought.

We even had a visit from a man that I believe was an angel, which my uncle Steve said that he believes was also an angel visiting us due to his story being strictly identical to my real-life experiences, something he'd not know about me as a normal human being.

My dad then went to the HealthSouth rehabilitation facility outside of Geisinger's main hospital unit, and my aunt Marci and uncle Dave brought us their RV to sleep in right outside of the rehabilitation center. My dad had to undergo excruciating physical, occupational, and speech therapies to help his entire left side of his body, all of which was numb due to the stroke he suffered. He couldn't walk, so he had to be in a wheelchair. He couldn't talk or eat properly. He couldn't feel his entire left side of his body. The doctors told him he'd not walk like he used to, and he'd never drive nor cook again. But they don't know my dad. My dad proved them wrong and months of rehabilitation, he is now driving, cooking, walking, and talking.

My dad finished his rehab, and halfway through his radiation treatments, he was pronounced cancer free. The best news of our lives. Something all cancer patients and their families dream to hear, that their loved one is in remission and all cancer cells are stabilized. My dad had to continue the radiation until the cycle was completed, to which he finished on my 28th birthday. The best birthday gift of my life was celebrating my 28th birthday on December 6, 2016 with the date my dad had his very last radiation treatment. Afterwards, we celebrated my birthday and my dad's last radiation treatment (while being cancer free) at the Mineshaft Café in Ashland, Pennsylvania, to which the owner, who is a good friend of my dad's, gave us both a free cake (me for my birthday and my dad for kicking cancer's ass).

My dad began his chemotherapy treatments via a pill and he then started the Optune Device, which is a device used to electromagnetically kill any dividing cancer cells in the brain that attempt to reform the tumor.

November 2017 saw the release of *Christ Defeats Cancer*, to which currently became a New York Times Best Selling novel, and as of the publication of the biographical novel, my dad remained cancer free. However, does that mean he's still cancer free? You will have to continue reading to find out. But before going into more of my dad's continuation and progression on his battle with Glioblastoma, why don't we give an in-depth, detailed, and analytical diagnostic report on this dreaded, deadly disease.

Once you find out what Glioblastoma is and does, you'll look at my dad just like I do, a hero, an inspiration, and a fighting survivor. Someone who is so brave to battle such a formidable foe. But something that isn't going to win because with Christ on your side, cancer itself stands no chance. We know *Christ Defeated Cancer*, but now let's find out what cancer Christ did defeat. Let's find out what cancer that Christ is obliterating when we go into round two with Glioblastoma. We're about to go into the knockout round: *Christ Defeats Cancer 2: The Battle Continues*.

CHAPTER 1: SATAN'S CURSE

For those who know, Satan is the evil one. The one against Jesus. The one that steals, kills, and destroys. He is the one that will do what he can to cause pain, torment, agony, sickness, fear, and disease. Satan is the one that causes the growth of tumors, the spreading of cancer, and the thoughts in your mind that makes you think the worst. In retrospect, if you come to Jesus then miracles are witnessed. Jesus doesn't cause the tumors to grow. He may allow them to progress, but if you come and seek him, then you will be able to witness the miracles like my dad had and my family has witnessed.

My faith was being tested when my dad was first diagnosed with stage four of Glioblastoma. I lost faith when we thought we were going to lose him. However, the miracle I had witnessed, which allowed my dad to ultimately defeat brain cancer in the first-round battle, my faith was restored. You must believe in Jesus and have the ultimate faith to get through the hardships of life. But what exactly is faith? As Saint Augustine said, "Faith is to believe what you do not see; the reward of this faith is to see what you believe."

The thing not really discussed in *Christ Defeats Cancer* was exactly what the curse Satan placed upon my dad and there was a reason for this. I wanted to focus on my dad's recovery, healing, and restoration, and not necessarily on the disease that Satan has caused. After all, Christ did defeat cancer. However, there are people wondering that if Christ defeated cancer in the first book, how is there a sequel to it. The first book is titled *Christ Defeats Cancer* **NOT** *Christ Defeated Cancer*. The healing process is just that…a process. Christ did defeat cancer the first round of the battle, and as with any cancer battle, the battle does indeed continue until Christ 100 percent defeats cancer. We believe, speak, and acknowledge my dad's healing, and it is up to our Lord and Savior, Jesus Christ, to do that and until he does, the battle will continue until the ultimate restoration of healing with all cancer cells and traces of Glioblastoma being obliterated from all MRI's.

The different of adding Glioblastoma into *Christ Defeats Cancer 2: The Battle Continues* is to show what kind of coward Satan is to cast upon his curse onto my dad and allow him to continue tormenting and torturing this dreaded cancer onto my dad. It is time that Satan is exposed and how to do this is to allow the revelation of Satan and Glioblastoma, so we can have followers of Jesus to become aware of this aggressive form of brain cancer, so we can help find the ultimate career, which can only happen through Jesus Christ himself.

So, that brings me to my next point: what exactly is stage four Glioblastoma? Glioblastoma is the most aggressive and deadliest form of cancer known to man and is located in either the brain or spine. It is extremely rare in the United States of America and has roughly less than 200,000 cases per year in the United States. This cancer is incurable (otherwise terminal in the natural world; curable through Jesus Christ of course), however, treatments can and most certainly do help those seeking it.

In order to treat Glioblastoma, there are the options of surgery, radiation, chemotherapy, and other types of treatments can be available, if recommended by the neurologist taking care of that patient. This type of tumor grows and spreads rapidly, often creating pressure. The symptoms and warning signs of suffering from stage four of Glioblastoma, include headaches, nausea, drowsiness, blurred vision, personality changes, and seizures, most of which my dad had, and requires a CT scan and/or MRI to determine the proper diagnosis.

Glioblastoma is the type of cancer, that with surgery, is unable to be removed completely via surgery. Even with surgery, regrowth of the cancer is probable and most likely will happen in the natural. However, we who have faith know the truth of Isaiah 53:5, "By his stripes we are healed." What that means is that Jesus is the ultimate physician. He gives the wisdom to the doctors and nurses on Earth, but it is Jesus who heals all wounds and is Jesus who cures all infectious and incurable diseases and cancers. And the moment he was abused and beaten on the way to the cross and up to the moment he took his final breath on said cross, he sacrificed himself to die for our sins, which led to the ultimate resurrection on Easter Sunday, three days after his crucifixion.

We were grateful to have the doctors we have had at Geisinger Medical Center in Danville, Pennsylvania. From Dr. Toms, who has done the brain surgery on my dad back in September 2016 and wrote the foreword to *Christ Defeats Cancer* to Dr. Turner and finally to Dr. Gatson, who came from the cancer institute in Texas to take care of my dad's battle with this horrid illness and has written the foreword to this book, *Christ Defeats Cancer 2: The Battle Continues*. We have been so blessed for our amazing physicians and neurologists, and in the end, it is the ultimate physician, Jesus Christ, who prevails in taking care of, managing, and obliterating Glioblastoma, not just from my father, but from existence.

The thing about Glioblastoma and its formation is due to cells specifically known as astrocytes. These astrocytes support the nerve cells. My dad just turned 56 years on August 12, 2018 and is quite young, however, Glioblastoma occurs at any age, but more often in older adults. It seems to be people in their 50s that tend to attract the tumor more than any other age group, at least from my own personal viewpoints from what I, myself, personally researched, read, and experienced.

With the treatments that I have previously mentioned, they'll slow the progression of the cancer and reduce the signs and symptoms, but without Jesus' will and supernatural power, Glioblastoma (also known as Glioblastoma Multiforme) is incurable, which means it is an inevitable fatal and terminal form of brain cancer. But those with faith in the superior higher power of the Lord, Jesus Christ, will have the ultimate defeat of Satan's curse known as Glioblastoma and Jesus will be the one to have the final laugh when he sends Satan to the bottomless pit to burn for eternity, along with Glioblastoma and any other cancer known to man. Because those who are reading this, bear witness to triumph. Say with me together that "By His stripes we are healed."

Let's end the discussion and lecture regarding Satan's curse of Glioblastoma, along with any other cancer in prayer. Say with me, "Father God, thank you for not just healing my father, Scott George McCoy, but every person on this planet who is or was battling cancer. Father God, please allow those currently consumed with curable or incurable cancers, as well as those currently in remission from their cancer to be healed by your supernatural touch. Father God, please obliterate each and every cancer cell that is in the body, blood, veins, organs, or any other aspects of the human anatomy because we confess that by your stripes we are healed. We say this in the loving and nurturing name of our Lord and Savior, Jesus Christ. Amen."

Saying such a prayer will make us in agreement that Glioblastoma and all other cancers are now at the mercy of the feet of Jesus. And I'm speaking to all the cancers, tumors, growths, cysts, and anything else that can grow and spread into a terminally-related illness, YOU WILL BOW TO THE FEET OF THE LAMB AND YOU WILL PERISH INTO THE FIERY DEPTHS OF HELL WITH YOUR MAKER, SATAN. Thank you, Lord Jesus, for this confession and restoration of health you have given those with such a battle and Satan's curse he has spawned since the moment he wreaked havoc on Earth for Jesus' children. We can now officially confession the healing hands of Jesus and that now cancer is destroyed, obliterated, and cured!

CHAPTER 2: LIVING WITH AFFLICTION

As those who remember, the past year and some months after my dad's original diagnosis with Glioblastoma have been a hard task to manage. If my dad never had the stroke two days after surgery, he'd not have been in such a horrible predicament. Not that it is a bad thing on us having to cater to him and help him out with anything he needs, but I know my own father, and he loves independence. It drives him insane having to sit around and get back to himself. He hates having people taking turns watching him or even drive him around from place to place. However, within due time, he got back a lot of his mobility and functionality. He was able to cook, drive, walk, talk, clean, or do anything he used to do, just not like he used to. He wasn't at 100 percent; however, he was darn close to it.

September 14, 2016 was the moment that changed not just my dad's life, but my life, my mom's life, and my entire family's lives forever. The moment my dad was diagnosed with brain cancer. In November 2017, *Christ Defeats Cancer* was published and did amazing in the selling department. Family, friends, and even strangers purchased the book, either directly from me or from Amazon itself. I even had people come to visit me and buy a book directly from me at select book signings, both people I know and strangers alike, and it was nice to see people that shared interest in a miraculous story regarding my father. I am always honored to discuss my dad's cancer battle and miraculous recovery and ultimate defeat through our Lord and Savior, Jesus Christ.

My dad was pronounced one-year cancer free around Thanksgiving of 2017. A blessing for sure when we first were told of his cancer free diagnosis the prior year and something to be thankful for. Every year on Thanksgiving, we celebrate my dad's cancer remission, even though the cancer he has is classified as "incurable" and we always have a reason to be thankful on this very day.

Then came Christmas 2017. My dad got to spend and live to see another Christmas with my mom and I, as well as our family. I remember when this first happened back in September, I thought that my dad wouldn't live to see Thanksgiving or even Christmas that year. Not only has he got to live and see those holidays, he got to cook, he was able to unwrap his gifts, and he was able to enjoy the holidays. It's amazing that a major brain surgery, on top of a life-threatening stroke, although it affected him drastically, he was able to get back to normal a few months after the fact.

He managed to get through some excruciating physical, occupational, and speech therapy. But in doing so, with tons of hard work to get back to the man he used to be, was discharged from inpatient treatments a month after receiving surgery. In return, he had to do outpatient therapies, but he did amazing with that as well and now look at him! He's back to the man he once was, and nothing'll stop him from being there for his wife, son, and family.

My dad gets his MRI's every two months so that if any tumor regrowth occurs that they'll be able to catch it in time. My dad is a strong man. A fighter for sure. I remember he always had his MRI's when I was working at Computer Software Incorporated. I worked there from November 2016 (a few months after his surgery and stroke, of course) to September 2017. It's funny because I could never focus, think, nor work because I was concerned with the pending MRI results. It was always that day too, as every other day I was fine. But it was due to the love I have for my father and the genuine human emotion of being concerned for a loved one. It was always my imagination and mind playing tricks on me. Or more like Satan putting the emotion of fear into my body. But the MRI's always turned out just fine.

A few months after the ultimate release of the strongly written and powerful testimonial of *Christ Defeats Cancer*, my dad started to have regrowth in his brain on a regularly scheduled MRI. There were just three little blobs shown on the MRI which indicated the tumor starting its progression process. Those three blobs of cancer regrowth were easily able to be obliterated with one thirty-minute radiation treatment.

Thankfully when the tumor was starting to regrow my dad didn't need to get any surgical procedures on the brain. I remember it like it was yesterday when my dad was getting brain surgery. It was God awful! The hours and hours of waiting…six hours to be exact. Waiting for the unknown. Praying for a positive outcome. Having hope and faith in the Lord to heal my dad and allow for a successful surgery. Thankfully that all came to fruition. And he didn't need another surgery roughly a year and a half later when regrowth of this curse Satan has cast started. It was small, minor, and easily manageable to be obliterated with radiation. And in the end, dad was back to his stabled self: cancer/tumor free.

The living with affliction is an exhausting, draining ordeal. It's the aftermath, or the after effect if you will, of the surgery, stroke, radiation, chemotherapy, and even the Optune device he wears that makes things so complicated.

It does so much to the brain, not necessarily damage, but just affects the brain drastically to the point that you sometimes get side effects, including, but not limited to memory loss, loss of balance, confusion, numbness, etc. But thankfully for my dad, even with some side effects, the first year and a half or so after this nightmare began seemed to improve more and more and the setbacks were minimal and easily maintainable.

Almost two years to the anniversary date and onward, we had a big setback. The first in the healing and recovery process. We can and will get through it together as a family, but it is a time that we reached out to our Lord and Savior, Jesus Christ, and began to pray for yet another amazing feat of strength on behalf of my dad through the Lord's supernatural and holy powers of healing and restoration.

CHAPTER 3: EXTENSIVE REHABILITATION

My dad, after having the three blobs of cancer cells that began look aggressive on an MRI removed, was doing great. A few more months would be two years since he was initially diagnosed with this horrid curse of Satan's known as Glioblastoma.

In a June 2018 MRI, Dr. Gatson noticed some formation in the brain that they weren't too concerned with and decided to keep an eye on it and see if it grows and stays the same size in the August 2018 MRI. Thing is, if it stays the same, it is most likely just a scarring from radiation. If it grows, it is ultimately another aggressive part of the tumor trying to regrow itself.

My dad was at Boy Scout Camp near the end of July 2018. About midweek, roughly Wednesday, he called my mom and told her that he lost complete feeling in his left leg and can barely walk on it. We kind of figured it was just something normal as one of his side effects for the chemo pill he takes is numbness of the limbs (legs, feet, arms, and hands).

Three weeks have passed, and he still had no feeling in his left leg, and he was compensating to move by using only his right leg. Granted, my dad never really had feeling in his left leg, he at least was able to move it and use it to walk properly. But now, he is unable to walk using his left leg. However, a few weeks later it has gotten worse.

Soon after he was using his right leg to compensate for his left, he was starting to get massive joint pain, primarily in his right hip. Soon after, my mom and dad, along with my aunt Lou Ann and uncle Kirk, were on a day trip to the Sands Casino in Bethlehem, Pennsylvania. They were on their way home from an overnight outing and stopped to eat at Cracker Barrel. My dad suddenly fell. It turned out to be a loss of feeling in his right leg. Like what? You just said he couldn't walk on his left leg, but now his right leg is unable to be used? Exactly! My parents, aunt, and uncle rushed home, my uncle Steve came to my house, and we all rushed my dad to the Geisinger Medical Center in Danville.

They kept him overnight in the main hospital unit in the Neurology wing of the hospital and checked what was going on. They did an MRI and there we have it. He apparently had excessive swelling in his brain and they were unable to determine if there was any tumor regrowth due to the amount of swelling covering the brain. I was terrified, but I still had my faith in the Lord, Jesus Christ, and his supernatural power to heal my dad and make us pass this hurdle as well.

My uncle Steve knew for a fact that this was not the end for my dad though. Not just by faith, but by his powerful testimonies through his theological visions he obtained from the Lord, Jesus Christ. Some visions my uncle had through these past few months or so of my dad's inability to walk include:

- ➢ A vision of the Holy Spirit releasing fire into the cavity of my dad's skull. The fire was touching different areas of the upper parts of my dad's brain.
- ➢ A vision of a well-lit candlestick inside my dad's skull. The flame was strong and bright. My uncle Steve sensed the candlestick as a symbol of God's anointing on my dad, as well as my dad's testimony to the goodness of the Lord Jesus.

> ➢ A vision of the Holy Spirit releasing an increase of light into my dad's cranial cavity to the point that it was complete filled. My uncle Steve sensed the words "Walking by faith and not by sight" and "To be worldly minded brings death, but to be spiritually minded brings life and peace."
> ➢ A vision of Jesus as the Lion of the tribe of Judah. As a lion, Jesus was licking various parts of my dad's brain. Saliva contains primarily water. My uncle Steve sensed Jesus was applying Living Water to my dad's brain tissue and its surrounding areas. My uncle, my mom, and myself have prayed with my dad to petition for our chief intercessor Lord Jesus to continue to prowl around like a Lion in my dad's cranial cavity.

They were such powerful visions the Lord Jesus gave to my uncle and prophesized among my dad's health with his battle of brain cancer, also known as the curse Satan had unleashed upon my dad, otherwise known as Glioblastoma. And ultimately we pray for and truly believe in the ultimate power of the Lord Jesus that he'll heal my dad and allow the worldly medical staff and brain cancer researchers to obtain the ability to find a cure for this horrid disease so my dad, among many, many others suffering from Satan's wicked curse to be healed, cured, and manifesting in the glory of the Lord.

Upon being told about the swelling he has in his brain, on top of not knowing if there is potential tumor regrowth due to the fact that the swelling is so excessive, they figured the best bet was to put my dad on steroids which'll shrink the swelling, as well as send him over to HealthSouth, which is the rehabilitation facility that

Geisinger owns, so he can have the proper rehab to get him walking again.

Upon being transferred to HealthSouth via a shuttle, he was worked hard. He was given extensive physical and occupational therapies by the best therapists in the industry. He was eventually walking again, with help from either a cane or a walker, whatever he has chosen was the best to use when he wanted to go somewhere and do something. He rang the bell at HealthSouth, and he has just finished his second time at the facility. For those who do not remember, he had his first time there after he sustained the stroke post-brain surgery almost two years prior.

It was the beginning of September, and my dad started new therapies known as immunotherapy which consisted of Avastin, which he would get every two weeks. The Avastin would strangle, or smother for a lack of a better word, the blood supply to the cancerous parts of the brain, which the treatment would be set to target. The old saying goes, "Tumors love blood. Cancer loves blood. Blood feeds into the tumor and, as such, will grow in size when the blood hits the specified tumor cells."

With that said, the Avastin therapy would be stopping all blood flow and supply to that specific part of the brain where the cancer cells are located so the tumor doesn't regrow. In doing so, it may not cure the cancer and remove all the cells, however, it'll stall and stop the feeding of the tumor to a point in which it would not increase and would stabilize, and even, decrease the tumor. In retrospect, it also shrinks the swelling in the brain to which is the reasoning my dad was unable to walk. The steroids took down some of the swelling and the Avastin therapies will keep the swelling down and the tumor to the size of a puny, little pebble.

My dad would do the Avastin therapy as an outpatient treatment at the Knapper Clinic, which is in the vicinity Geisinger in Danville. Upon doing this, he would also have at home physical and occupational therapy. He had physical therapy a lot longer than he had occupational therapy. His physical therapist's name was Tammy and she did amazing with my dad. The insurance only allowed my dad to continue the physical therapy for ninety days, and afterwards, he'd have to wait another ninety days until he was able to begin the therapy again.

As my dad continued the at home physical therapy, which he had only one day per week, Tammy had noticed something about my dad in the past few weeks. And what she had noticed scared both my mom and me. Something that made us think that we're on the verge of another setback.

CHAPTER 4: TWO YEARS LATER

September 2016 was an emotional for not just my mom and I, but also for our entire family as it marked two years of one of the worst days of our lives. It marked two years that my dad was diagnosed with Satan's curse known as Glioblastoma. But, we know deep down that my dad is cured, even if not pronounced cured by the medical staff. The reasoning we belief he is cured without a medical diagnosis is because the Lord our God, Jesus Christ, has simply foretold so.

As previously mentioned, Tammy noticed my dad declining during his at home physical therapy. He had an MRI at the end of October 2018 to which showed his tumor was extremely small and there was some swelling in the brain, but not that much of it.

Tammy awaited till we had the results of the MRI to tell my mom and I of what she has noticed, and since the MRI was unable to determine why my dad is not walking as he used to, Tammy decided to tell us that my dad has been declining the past few weeks, each week being worse than the last. Over the past three weeks of my dad doing the at home physical therapy, he gradually declined each passing week and Tammy thought she saw signs of him having a stroke, even if it was a mini stroke.

She assured us she is no doctor, but that there is something neurological happening that is not allowing the physical therapy to help him, but to decline his ability in moving. On top of this, my dad's blood pressure was through the roof. With massively high blood pressure and the fact he is unable to walk like he used to, with a steady declination of movement, what else could it be other than a stroke? So, Dr. Gatson had put my dad on blood pressure medication and it started to get his blood pressure down to a proper and appropriate level.

I remember I was scared beyond belief when I heard my mom crying upstairs randomly one morning. I went upstairs and there was my dad lying in my mom's arms and his eyes were closed. I thought my dad passed away and I didn't know what to do. I almost began to cry and hyperventilate. My dad then opened his eyes and told us he thinks that he is dying. This is a story I haven't told anyone, not even on Facebook, but it is something that I want to put in this book. It was the most horrifying moment of my life.

A few hours later my dad was back to normal, he was just having bad thoughts, flashbacks to his childhood, and figured that his time was ending. Thankfully that wasn't the case, but boy did it scare me. That is just one of the ways Satan works his demonic magic to make people think the worse is happening and nothing bad was happening at all.

All of us, even us as Christians, have negative thoughts and have Satan get into our minds because that is also called being human. But we must cast out Satan in the name of Jesus Christ from Nazareth who came in the flesh because we all know that Satan is terrified of our Lord, Jesus Christ.

I then took my dad to an Avastin treatment roughly a week later and they told us, after two hours of waiting in the waiting room, that they cannot do his therapy because he cannot walk, and they want to make sure that it wasn't something regarding his brain. So, as a safety protocol, I had to rush my dad over to the emergency room to which we were waiting for a long, long time.

I called my aunt Marci and she, along with her husband, my uncle Dave, met us at the emergency room. My mom was Christmas shopping with her best friend, Laura, and we told her to not bother coming up and we'll keep her informed. Granted, my mom just had surgery on her sciatica and she needed to get out and do her own thing and not worry about my dad like she has been the past two years. On top of the fact that she was roughly two hours away from the hospital, there was no point in her coming to the hospital now.

We got to the ER around 11:30 AM or so and we knew this would be a long, long day. There is no easy and quick wait in an emergency room waiting room. As the hours passed by, it was now 5:00 PM and I went up to the secretary, after asking how long of a wait it would be and telling them that we think my dad may have had a mini stroke. Last time I checked, a mini stroke is considered a major medical emergency and should be addressed right away, but as you have previously read, it was 5:00 PM and we have yet to be seen.

Upon reaching the secretary's desk for the second time, I lashed out at her for the extensive, uncalled for wait time, as my aunt Marci filed an online complaint through Geisinger's Website. We tell them we think my dad had a mini stroke, as my dad's blood pressure was even high at the triage, on top of not being able to walk, and we waited all this time.

My dad still laughs and makes fun of me, in a joking aspect, of how I yelled at the receptionist. I said something along the lines of, "This is getting ridiculous!

We have been waiting for more than five hours. If we are not seen in the next fifteen minutes, we're leaving!" My dad laughed and saw me seething, but to this day he jokes around saying, "The receptionist was probably like thank God. You were in a hospital, not a restaurant." Something I felt needed to be said at the time but thinking back it was a hospital and not a restaurant. They probably couldn't care less if we left or not as it was less wait time for others behind us.

There was even this one guy waiting in the emergency room and his blood pressure was low. He was yelling and complaining too with the wait time. They checked his blood pressure and it was still low. Mine and the rest of the room's blood pressure was probably sky high, but this poor man still couldn't get it up.

We finally got called back and they did a CT scan on my dad and all came back well and good. They decided it was best to keep him overnight due to safety concerns. I made sure this time everything was thoroughly checked and not just an MRI on his brain, which they did do and came back the same as his last MRI, which was a good thing. I made sure that he got an MRI of his spine to make sure there is nothing going wrong there, as well as any other tests they can do to make sure they find a source of his inability to walk.

The MRI of his spine and neck came back fine. There were no signs of cancer or any types of tumors, which was a huge sigh of relief. They also did a muscular test on his legs and he also passed that, which made us think why he cannot walk. His MRI of his brain is normal, the MRI of his spine and neck came back perfectly fine, and he has no pinched nerves or any type of issues in his muscles and nerves that operate his legs. So, what could be causing this.

Dr. Gatson investigated this and told us it is the disease, yes Satan's curse of Glioblastoma, itself. Glioblastoma is the culprit. She didn't expand in detail on what that meant, and we had no clue on what this could mean, yet. She did say that my dad is going back to HealthSouth, yes for a third time, and he'll have to get more physical and occupational rehabilitation to straighten out his walking inabilities, but this time we are going to make sure that he walks and doesn't have any more sets back.

After countless calls and appeals to the insurance company, with two denials from them, we were able to make sure they knew without a shadow of a doubt that they would pay for my dad's rehabilitation as it is medically necessary and there isn't anything they can say or do to prove this otherwise. I mean, for God sakes, my dad's primary neurologist is saying he needs this to be done and without a shadow of a doubt, my dad is getting the rehab he needs, and he was eventually approved upon the third appeal.

Before my dad was transferred over to HealthSouth, I surprised him and drove up to the hospital to visit him. He was so shocked. He looked at me and didn't budge. He must've thought he was seeing things. He then looked again and saw me. I came into his room, he was crying, and gave me a big hug. I saw some tears trickling down the side of his cheek as he was so excited and happy to see me, not even expecting my visit as it was a complete surprise for him that I had planned the night prior.

My dad's stay in Geisinger was going to be brief because in a few days' time, my dad was being transferred over to HealthSouth for the third and hopefully the last time for extensive rehabilitation to finally get my dad walking again.

CHAPTER 5: THE MANIFESTATION OF MOBILITY

My dad was finally transferred over to HealthSouth upon approval by the insurance company. It was funny because we knew he wouldn't be spending Thanksgiving with us, which marked two years to the day of being pronounced tumor free without regrowth and progression. My mom and I went down to my aunt Lou Ann and uncle Kirk's house for Thanksgiving and we ate our Thanksgiving feast together, along with my cousin Derek and his girlfriend, Marissa, as well as my nana.

After we finished eating, my mom and I, along with my uncle Kirk and aunt Lou Ann went to visit my dad and bring him a platter in the hospital. My aunt Lesley was in the parking lot waiting for us, and then my aunt Marci, uncle Dave, and my cousin Jennifer came up about an hour later. It was a nice surprise to see amazing family friends, Lynn and Rick, as they visited my dad on Thanksgiving as well, something none of us was aware of. Of course, Lynn and I had to get a selfie together.

Oh, and remember when I previously mentioned how my dad jokingly makes fun of my outburst in the emergency room towards the secretary? Well, he even told the story to everyone there visiting him on Thanksgiving, which had us all laughing since everyone knows how I am and how I react in the most dramatic way possible.

My dad later told me he was visited by the head boss at HealthSouth and he took my dad for a walk to assess how far he can walk before he gets tired out. Well, he gave us insights and it gave us a revelation on why my dad was not able to walk, despite all the MRIs and testing coming back good. He told us that Dr. Gatson is right about it being the disease causing the inability of walking, but he elaborated more to us than she has which gave us a greater insight on what has been happening to my dad.

He told us that the part of the brain where the disease is located is affecting his legs. That specific part of the brain needs retraining because it has literally forgotten how to walk. Each part of the brain represents specific parts of the body, including memory, arms, legs, etc. The part being affected in my dad's brain is his legs and he said that the continuing physical therapy would be focusing on retraining the brain to think to walk and not focusing on the muscular part of walking.

My dad had an Avastin treatment while in HealthSouth, so they shuttled him from HealthSouth to the Knapper Clinic. He waited for roughly two hours before receiving his treatment and ultimately came across an elderly lady who worked as a chaplain at the hospital. He told her what he was in the hospital for and how he had been suffering from Glioblastoma and how he wasn't even supposed to survive the stroke he sustained after surgery. The chaplain told my dad that he didn't die because the Lord isn't ready for him. The Lord still isn't ready for him she told my dad and continued saying that his work on Earth isn't done as the Lord plans on using my dad and his struggle as a testimony to the powerful and miraculous works of the Lord.

My dad told me that he doesn't care how long it takes to be released from HealthSouth, he just wants to walk out and not be wheeled out in a wheelchair. And boy is my dad ever motivated.

Here comes December 6, 2018, my 29th birthday. My dad's release date. My uncle Steve, my mom, and I all drove to HealthSouth to get my dad out of the hospital and bring him home. I remember it vividly, I kept getting happy birthday compliments from the fellow workers there because of my Santa Claus hat overlapped with a "Happy Birthday" tiara draped across it.

My dad got to ring the bell for the third time total and we were hoping that we don't have to go back to HealthSouth again. They are a nice facility, but not going back means that my dad is manifesting the mobility factor, meaning he is able to walk and do things on his own. The best part of this HealthSouth stay was the fact that my dad bent his left leg for the first time since July 2018. That was a huge accomplishment that we were so grateful to witness.

As the weeks progressed, my dad would continue to do at home therapies like he did before he was admitted to HealthSouth, including physical therapy with Tammy, occupational therapy with Richard, and speech therapy with Mary. Mary told me a story at one of my dad's visits during his speech therapy that was also classified as a miracle story.

She told us that she was diagnosed with breast cancer. She needed to have a double mastectomy to remove the breast tissue and the cancer cells that made home inside of it. She went to a prayer group and they laid hands upon her. They told her that they felt the cancer within her breasts had left her body and she was healed. She went in for the surgery and they found out that she had no more breast cancer and she only had a partial mastectomy.

I absolutely love hearing miracle stories because my family, personally, experienced one with my own father and seeing other's receiving a miracle to share with us is all part of God's plan and how he uses it to manifest healing, hope, and faith to others who just don't see the good happening and just the inevitable end. Just because the doctor tells you that you have a few days to live doesn't mean that you are on the brink of death. My dad was told the same, but over two years later and he is still alive and kicking. A cancer that is supposed to take your life in no more than two years has my dad going stronger than ever and the cancer hasn't even continued to grow, which has the doctors amazed, surprised, dumbfounded, and even relieved.

The Avastin and OPDIVO treatments are doing their job because my dad had another MRI the day after Christmas Day on December 26, 2018 and it was better than the last MRI he had. Everything was remaining stable, but some of the swelling in the brain was improved. When I say improved, I mean that some of the swelling was shrunk and not as large as it was in the prior MRI my dad had.

You must remember that doctors are just educated medical personnel. But our overall doctor who knows how to manifest complete healing is the good Lord himself, Jesus Christ. He is the ultimate healer and physician. He is the one that can manifest a full recovery and healing upon anyone, including my dad and you, the reader, and your family members. You must have faith, even if it is hard to do, and remember that "By Jesus' stripes, you are healed."

It may be hard to live solely by faith, as it was for me. But even though I was a Christian before everything that occurred with my dad, my faith was strengthened by seeing how the works of the Lord happened and how I witnessed a miracle right in front of my own two eyes. The fact that my prayers, my family's prayers, and the entire world's prayers have been answered, well that was a true miracle in and of itself. Seeing all my friends, family, and fans joining together and praying for my dad was a true miracle and the fact that those prayers were answered was the greatest gift I could've ever received. I mean, my dad even got a get well soon card back in 2016 from a fan of mine located in The Netherlands.

I thought I'd never spend another birthday or Christmas with my dad, but December 2018 was the third birthday and Christmas I got to spend with my dad since this all started. And in the present day, my dad is still doing great and going strong. His manifestation of mobility is still going strong.

His physical therapist, Tammy, was here on January 15, 2019 and she told us something we were so happy to hear, and I quote, "Scott is doing amazing and walking better than I have ever saw him walk and get around since I started with him in Fall 2018." That alone has us giving glory to God.

My cousin Derek has become my dad's caretaker. He helps my dad do exercises outside of his scheduled therapies. He helps him get around the house and do outside activities, like cleaning up. My dad even went upstairs, with help from myself and my cousin, of course, and he didn't fall, he was able to do it, and we were so proud of him accomplishing something of that magnitude. I have no clue how long it has been since my dad walked up and down steps, outside of his therapies at HealthSouth, of course.

Another accomplishment my dad did that had me so proud, as well as Tammy amazed, was the fact that he went into the laundry room by himself and did his own wash, then went to the bathroom and brushed his teeth. I haven't seen my dad since, so I obviously went to look for him. Here he was, sleeping in his bed. I usually have to help him into bed, or my mom has to help him get his legs up onto the bed, but he did it all by himself. An accomplishment that I am proud to tell anyone and everyone who wants to hear. My dad never was able to do that, but that time he knew he wanted to try and he did succeed.

So, my dad's manifestation of mobility has become increasingly strong. With a cancer, or Satan's curse if you will, that usually has a lifespan of two years at the most, has my dad going on almost two and a half years, and he is showing no signs of slowing down. You know why? Because my dad is strong. My dad is a fighter. And most importantly, my dad has Jesus Christ on his side.

If you or anyone you know is battling cancer, just remember that Jesus is real, and he'll help you when you need it. He'll give you the motivation, willpower, and strength to overcome the odds. He'll perform the manifestation of miracles in your life, if you surrender yourself to him, believe in him, have faith in him, and put your life and trust into him. You can do all things through Christ. You can overcome the odds. You can kneel to the feet of the Lamb because he is the one who can and will make your life easier to live.

Just remember, this isn't my story. I am the author writing about a miraculous story regarding my father. This is my father's testimony told through me and the Holy Spirit within me. And the Lord has brought me into your life to show you that all things are possible through him and that if you shall believe in him, you shall not perish, but have eternal life. Surrender yourself to Jesus because if you do, you too will have eternal life. You too will see true miracles. And you too will be healed.

Amen

BONUS CHAPTER: WHAT IS A MIRACLE?

The definition of a miracle is "a surprising and welcome event that is not explicable by natural or scientific laws and is therefore considered to be the work of a divine agency." Simply put, doctors cannot perform miracles, only a supernatural entity can do so. And this book is my dad's testimony written through the Holy Spirit within myself as an author to declare the works for the Lord and show that my dad is the true miracle that was performed by Jesus Christ himself.

In this bonus chapter, I am going to show you the times that miracles were performed and mentioned in the Bible to prove to you that, not only is my dad a miracle, but you can be too.

> "By faith in the name of Jesus, this man whom you see and know was made strong. It is Jesus' name and the faith that comes through him that has completely healed him, as you can all see."
>
> Acts 3:16

> "He is the one you praise; he is your God, who performed for you those great and awesome wonders you saw with your own eyes."
>
> Deuteronomy 10:21

"He said, 'If you listen carefully to the Lord your God and do what is right in his eyes, if you pay attention to his commands and keep all his decrees, I will not bring on you any of the diseases I brought on the Egyptians, for I am the Lord, who heals you.'"

Exodus 15:26

"What Jesus did here in Cana of Galilee was the first of the signs through which he revealed his glory; and his disciples believed in him."

John 2:11

"Jesus replied, 'What is impossible with man is possible with God.'"

Luke 18:27

"He replied, 'Because you have so little faith. Truly I tell you, if you have faith as small as a mustard seed, you can say to this mountain, 'Move from here to there,' and it will move. Nothing will be impossible for you.'"

Matthew 17:20

""'If you can'?' said Jesus. 'Everything is possible for one who believes.'"

Mark 9:23

"I will not venture to speak of anything except what Christ has accomplished through me in leading the Gentiles to obey God by what I have said and done. By the power of signs and wonders, through the power of the Spirit of God. So, from Jerusalem all the way around to Illyricum, I have fully proclaimed the gospel of Christ."
                                        Romans 15:18-19

"God did extraordinary miracles through Paul, so that even handkerchiefs and aprons that had touched him were taken to the sick, and their illnesses were cured, and the evil spirits left them."
                                        Acts 19:11-12

"But if I were you, I would appeal to God; I would lay my cause before him. He performs wonders that cannot be fathomed, miracles that cannot be counted."
                                        Job 5:8-9

"Now, Lord, consider their threats and enable your servants to speak your word with great boldness. Stretch out your hand to heal and perform signs and wonders through the name of your holy servant, Jesus. After they prayed, the place where they were meeting was shaken. And they were all filled with the Holy Spirit and spoke the word of God boldly."
                                        Acts 4:29-31

"And these signs will accompany those who believe: In my name, they will drive out demons; they will speak in new tongues; they will pick up snakes with their hands; and when they drink deadly poison, it will not hurt them at all; they will place their hands on sick people, and they will get well. After the Lord Jesus had spoken to them, he was taken up into Heaven and he sat at the right hand of God. Then, the disciples went out and preached everywhere, and the Lord worked with them and confirmed his word by the signs that accompanied it."

Mark 16:17-20

"And a woman was there who had been subject to bleeding for twelve years, but no one could heal her. She came up behind him and touched the edge of his cloak, and immediately her bleeding stopped. 'Who touched me?' Jesus asked. When they all denied it, Peter said, 'Master, the people are crowding and pressing against you.' But Jesus said, 'Someone touched me; I know that power has gone out from me.' Then the woman, seeing that she could not go unnoticed came trembled and fell at his feet. In the presence of all the people, she told why she had touched him and how she had been instantly healed. Then he said to her, 'Daughter, your faith has healed you. Go in peace.'"

Luke 8:43-48

EPILOGUE

Thank you to everyone who has purchased *Christ Defeats Cancer* and for everyone who has continued to support myself and my family by purchasing its sequel, *Christ Defeats Cancer 2: The Battle Continues.*

The goal of this book is to not make a profit, although I do as it is my job as a writer to profit from my hard work, research, and communication with third party sources, including Dr. Gatson and the Geisinger legal team in regards to releasing confidential information of my dad's medical records, is primarily to show everyone that the Lord Jesus has helped my dad, as well as my family, cope with this huge downfall of life known as disease, or more specifically cancer. Our goal with these books are to educate people on what Christ has done for us and give hope and inspiration to those in similar situations to know not all is lost.

I always hear in regard to this book's title, "Well, Christ didn't save my family member from cancer" or "My family is religious, but why did God spare your family member but not help mine?" The simple answer is, "I don't got the answer to those questions. I am simply spreading my family's situation and how we personally have seen these miracles happen and to let everyone know that God has a purpose for everyone's lives and everyone's time is set before we're born. But just because God didn't spare your family member's life doesn't mean he abandoned them. It simply means their time on Earth has been fulfilled.

On a totally different subject, let's speak about this book and a special significance for it. *Christ Defeats*

Cancer 2: The Battle Continues was published on September 14, 2019. This is a special and significant date as it marks three years (36 months) of my dad's initial diagnosis with Glioblastoma. A terminal cancer we were told (post-stroke) would give him only 16 months of survival, which has now made 36 months and counting. But it doesn't end there…

After speaking with Dr. Gatson in regard to the foreword, she was gracious enough to inform me that my dad is one of a very few select people with Glioblastoma to survive for over the life expectancy of 16 months. He is past the 36-month mark and is in the five percent of survival for longer than 1 ½ years. The doctors are still baffled by how well my dad is doing after this battle with brain cancer and how he is not showing any bad signs from his immunotherapy treatments. They are shocked at how well his body is holding up, as most people don't make it this long, and since it is still working, they want to continue with the treatments that work for him.

With that said, everything in this book, from Dr. Gatson's foreword to the written testimonial from myself in regard to my experiences during the past three years of dealing with this excruciatingly exhausting journey is of my dad's progress. The treatments, medications, or outcomes of what has happened with my dad these past three years may or may not work for others going through the same thing. Remember, every person is different and what works for my dad may not work for you or your loved ones.

One thing to take away from these past three years is that the power of prayer works and is a super powerful thing. Keep praying to the Lord, develop a close relationship with him, and just have faith, hope, and belief in God and that he'll ease your pain and help provide medical care to yourself or your loved ones. Jesus Christ is the ultimate healer and the most knowledgeable physician there is, so he is the one to put your trust and faith into. He will provide the answers and comfort to your prayers. Believe in Jesus, HE IS the answer!

MCCOY MEMORIAL

Rest in peace to all my dad's side of the family that have crossed over into the Kingdom of Heaven to be with our Lord and Savior Jesus Christ

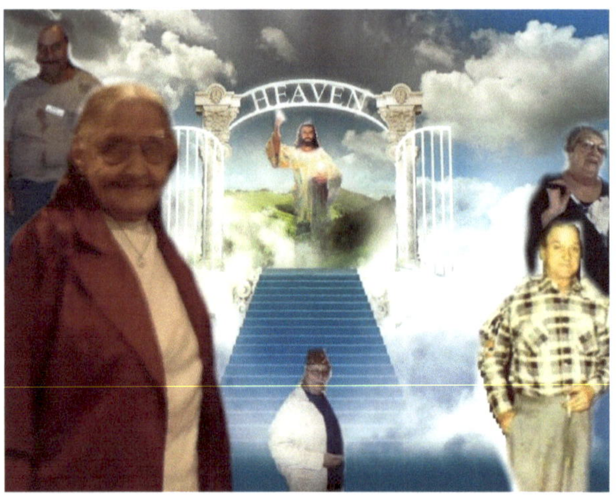

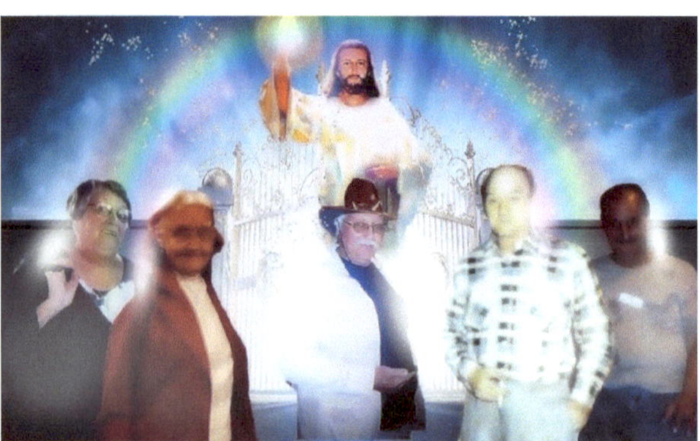

CONTACT

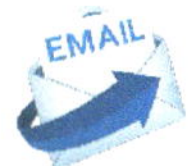 smccoyauthor@gmail.com

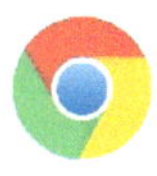 www.smccoyauthor.com

SOCIAL MEDIA LOUNGE

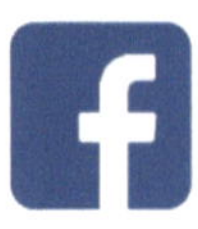 www.facebook.com/smccoyauthor

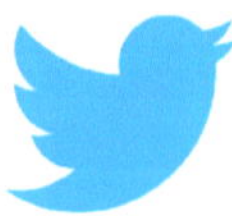 www.twitter.com/smccoyauthor

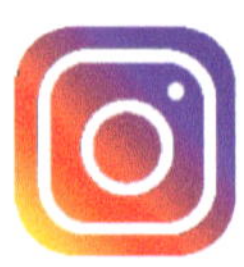 www.instagram.com/smccoyauthor

www.ingramcontent.com/pod-product-compliance
Lightning Source LLC
Chambersburg PA
CBHW040227240726
48664CB00001B/34